Book Title: "The Ultimate Guide to Anti-Inflammatory Foods For Gout"...

Gout, often referred to as the "disease of kings," has plagued humanity for centuries. It is a type of inflammatory arthritis characterized by sudden, severe attacks of pain, swelling, and redness in the joints, most commonly the big toe. While gout can be excruciatingly painful, it is also highly manageable, and one of the most effective ways to do so is through dietary choices....

This comprehensive guide is dedicated to exploring the world of anti-inflammatory foods and how they can be a game-changer in managing gout. We will delve into the intricate details of gout, uncover the role of inflammation in this condition, and provide you with a step-by-step plan to embrace an anti-inflammatory diet....

Gout is not an ailment that can be taken lightly. It affects your daily life, mobility, and overall well-being. But with the right knowledge and a commitment to making healthier food choices, you can significantly reduce the frequency and intensity of gout attacks....

In the chapters that follow, we will break down the science behind gout and inflammation, explore the wealth of anti-inflammatory foods available to you, and offer practical advice on how to incorporate them into your meals. Whether you're new to gout or have been battling it for years, this book is your ultimate resource for understanding and combatting this painful condition....

So, let's embark on this enlightening journey towards a pain-free, gout-free life. Chapter by chapter, we will empower you with the knowledge and tools needed to make informed decisions about your diet and health. Welcome to "The Ultimate Guide to Anti-Inflammatory Foods For Gout." Your path to relief starts here....

Chapter 1: Understanding Gout: Causes and Symptoms...

Gout, often considered a disease of excess, has been historically associated with indulgence in rich foods and alcoholic beverages. However, the reality is more complex. Gout is a form of inflammatory arthritis caused by the accumulation of uric acid crystals in the joints. In this chapter, we will explore the intricacies of gout, its causes, and the telltale signs and symptoms that set it apart from other health issues....

The Root Cause of Gout...

At the heart of gout lies a substance called uric acid. This chemical compound is a natural byproduct of the breakdown of purines, which are found in many of the foods we consume. Normally, uric acid dissolves in the blood and is excreted through the kidneys. However, in individuals with gout, this process is disrupted....

The Four Stages of Gout...

Asymptomatic Hyperuricemia: The first stage is characterized by elevated uric acid levels in the blood but no outward symptoms....

Acute Gout (Gouty Arthritis): This is the stage where the infamous gout attacks occur. Sharp, intense pain, swelling, and redness in the joints, often in the big toe, are the hallmarks of this phase....

Interval or Intercritical Gout: After the acute attack subsides, a person enters the intercritical phase, which is symptom-free. However, uric acid levels remain high, and without intervention, further attacks are likely....

Chronic Tophaceous Gout: If left untreated, gout can progress to the chronic tophaceous stage, marked by the development of tophi—painful deposits of uric acid crystals—under the skin, in joints, and even in organs....

Identifying Gout: Symptoms to Watch For...

Gout presents with several distinctive symptoms, making it relatively easy to diagnose. The key features include:...

Sudden Onset: Gout attacks typically come on suddenly, often in the middle of the night....

Intense Pain: The pain is usually excruciating, and the affected joint is tender, swollen, and warm to the touch....

Limited Mobility: Due to the pain and swelling, movement of the affected joint becomes severely restricted....

Redness: The joint may turn red or purplish during an attack....

Duration: Gout attacks can last anywhere from a few days to several weeks....

Understanding these symptoms is crucial, as an early diagnosis and proper management can prevent further damage and improve your quality of life. In the following chapters, we will explore how dietary changes, including the incorporation of anti-inflammatory foods, can play a pivotal role in gout management....

Chapter 2: The Role of Inflammation in Gout...

In the quest to manage gout effectively, it's essential to understand the role inflammation plays in this condition. Inflammation is the body's natural response to injury, infection, or harmful substances. However, when it becomes chronic, as is the case with gout, it can exacerbate the symptoms and contribute to long-term joint damage....

The Inflammatory Cascade...

Gout is often referred to as an "autoinflammatory" disease because it involves the body's immune system mistakenly attacking its tissues. In the case of gout, the trigger is the presence of uric acid crystals in the joints. Here's how the inflammatory cascade unfolds:...

Uric Acid Crystals: When uric acid levels in the blood become too high, the excess uric acid can form crystals. These crystals are sharp and needle-like, making them a potent irritant when they come into contact with joint tissues....

Immune Response: The body's immune system recognizes these crystals as foreign invaders and mounts an immune response. White blood cells and inflammatory molecules rush to the affected joint to eliminate the perceived threat....

Inflammation: The influx of white blood cells and the release of inflammatory molecules, such as cytokines, leads to inflammation. This inflammatory response is what causes the redness, swelling, and pain characteristic of gout attacks....

Secondary Damage: In addition to the immediate discomfort, this chronic inflammation can lead to secondary damage in the joints. Over time, the repeated cycles of inflammation can erode joint cartilage and bone....

The Vicious Cycle...

What makes gout particularly challenging is the cyclical nature of its attacks. Each gout episode can lead to more uric acid crystals forming in the joint, which, in turn, triggers further inflammation. This vicious cycle can result in more frequent and severe attacks if left unmanaged....

Anti-Inflammatory Foods as a Solution...

Now that we understand the inflammatory component of gout, it becomes evident why anti-inflammatory foods are a valuable tool in managing this condition. By incorporating foods that reduce inflammation into your diet, you can potentially break the cycle of gout attacks and mitigate their impact....

In the chapters ahead, we will explore a wide range of anti-inflammatory foods, from fruits and vegetables to lean proteins and spices, all of which can help reduce inflammation and improve your overall health. We'll provide detailed information on how these foods work and offer practical tips on incorporating them into your daily meals....

Remember, the goal isn't just to manage gout; it's to live a life free from the debilitating pain and limitations it imposes. Armed with knowledge about the inflammatory aspects of gout and the power of anti-inflammatory foods, you are well on your way to achieving that goal....

In the following chapters, we will delve deeper into specific dietary choices and strategies to help you take control of your gout and enjoy a higher quality of life....

Chapter 3: Diet and Lifestyle Factors in Gout Management...

To effectively manage gout and harness the power of anti-inflammatory foods, it's crucial to consider not only what you eat but also how your lifestyle impacts this condition. In this chapter, we will explore the interconnectedness of diet and lifestyle in gout management and provide you with practical guidance to make meaningful changes....

The Holistic Approach to Gout Management...

Gout is not just about what you put on your plate; it's also about the choices you make every day. Lifestyle factors can either exacerbate or alleviate gout symptoms. Here are some key aspects to consider:...

Hydration: Staying well-hydrated is essential for gout management. Adequate water intake helps flush excess uric acid from your system, reducing the risk of crystal formation in the joints....

Alcohol Consumption: Alcohol, particularly beer and spirits, can increase uric acid levels and trigger gout attacks. Moderation is key, and some individuals may need to avoid alcohol altogether....

Weight Management: Maintaining a healthy weight is vital for gout sufferers. Excess body weight can lead to higher uric acid levels and increased pressure on joints, making gout attacks more likely and more painful....

Exercise: Regular physical activity can aid in weight management and improve overall joint health. However, it's essential to choose activities that are gentle on the joints to avoid injury during gout attacks....

Medications: Depending on the severity of your gout and your individual risk factors, your healthcare provider may prescribe medications to manage uric acid levels. These medications work in tandem with dietary and lifestyle changes....

A Balanced Diet for Gout...

While anti-inflammatory foods are a cornerstone of gout management, it's also essential to maintain a balanced diet that meets your nutritional needs. Here are some dietary considerations:...

Portion Control: Overeating, especially foods high in purines (such as organ meats and shellfish), can contribute to gout attacks. Controlling portion sizes is key to gout-friendly eating....

Nutrient-Rich Foods: A diet rich in vitamins, minerals, and antioxidants supports overall health. Incorporate a variety of fruits, vegetables, whole grains, and lean proteins into your meals....

Limit Sugar and Processed Foods: High-sugar and highly processed foods can promote inflammation. Reducing or eliminating them from your diet is beneficial....

Moderate Purine Intake: While purines are found in many foods, not all purine-containing foods are created equal. Some are more likely to trigger gout attacks than others. We will explore this further in later chapters....

Personalized Gout Management...

Gout is a highly individualized condition. What works for one person may not work for another. Therefore, it's essential to work closely with your healthcare provider and possibly a registered dietitian to develop a personalized gout management plan that considers your unique needs, preferences, and medical history....

In the upcoming chapters, we will delve into the specifics of anti-inflammatory foods, providing you with a wealth of information and practical tips to make informed dietary choices. We will also explore gout-friendly recipes that not only support your health but also tantalize your taste buds. Together, we will empower you to take control of your gout and live a healthier, pain-free life....

Chapter 4: Anti-Inflammatory Foods: A Comprehensive Overview...

Now that we've laid the foundation for understanding gout and its connection to inflammation, it's time to dive headfirst into the world of anti-inflammatory foods. In this chapter, we will provide a comprehensive overview of these foods, helping you build a solid understanding of how they can benefit your gout management journey....

The Power of Anti-Inflammatory Foods...

Anti-inflammatory foods are those that possess natural properties to reduce inflammation in the body. They are packed with vitamins, minerals, antioxidants, and phytochemicals that combat the inflammatory response. When incorporated into your diet, these foods can help alleviate gout symptoms and improve your overall health....

Here's a broad overview of some key categories of anti-inflammatory foods:...

Fruits: Fruits are rich in vitamins, minerals, and antioxidants that help combat inflammation. Berries, cherries, citrus fruits, and apples are particularly beneficial for gout sufferers....

Vegetables: Leafy greens, broccoli, cauliflower, and colorful vegetables like bell peppers and tomatoes are excellent choices. They provide essential nutrients and fiber that support a healthy inflammatory response....

Whole Grains: Opt for whole grains like oats, quinoa, brown rice, and whole wheat bread over refined grains. These grains are packed with fiber and nutrients that promote anti-inflammatory effects....

Lean Proteins: Incorporate lean sources of protein such as poultry, fish (especially fatty fish like salmon), and plant-based proteins like tofu and legumes. These proteins provide necessary amino acids without the excess purines found in red meats....

Nuts and Seeds: Almonds, walnuts, flaxseeds, and chia seeds are rich in healthy fats and antioxidants that have anti-inflammatory properties....

Herbs and Spices: Turmeric, ginger, garlic, and cinnamon are known for their potent anti-inflammatory effects. They can be used to add flavor to your dishes while promoting joint health....

Gout and Purines: What You Need to Know...

While most anti-inflammatory foods are excellent choices for gout sufferers, it's essential to be mindful of purines. Purines are natural compounds found in many foods and are broken down into uric acid in the body. Excessive purine intake can exacerbate gout symptoms. Here's how to navigate this:...

Low-Purine Foods: Some anti-inflammatory foods are low in purines and can be safely incorporated into your gout-friendly diet. These include most fruits and vegetables....

Moderate-Purine Foods: Certain foods, like beans and legumes, contain moderate levels of purines but are generally safe for gout sufferers when consumed in moderation....

High-Purine Foods: Foods high in purines, such as organ meats, shellfish, and red meat, should be consumed sparingly or avoided altogether....

In the upcoming chapters, we will take a closer look at each category of anti-inflammatory foods, providing you with detailed information, practical tips, and mouthwatering recipes to make these foods a regular part of your diet. Remember, the key to gout management is not just what you avoid but also what you embrace on your plate....

Chapter 5: Fruits That Fight Inflammation...

Fruits are nature's gifts, brimming with vitamins, minerals, antioxidants, and fiber that make them essential components of an anti-inflammatory diet for gout. In this chapter, we'll explore various fruits that not only tantalize your taste buds but also help combat inflammation and support your journey toward gout management....

Berries: A Bounty of Antioxidants...

Berries are some of the most potent anti-inflammatory fruits available. They are rich in antioxidants like anthocyanins, quercetin, and vitamin C, which play a crucial role in reducing inflammation and protecting your cells from oxidative stress....

Blueberries: Blueberries are nutritional powerhouses known for their high antioxidant content.

They have been linked to reduced inflammation and improved cognitive function....

Strawberries: Strawberries are not only delicious but also rich in vitamin C and manganese, both of which contribute to anti-inflammatory effects....

Cherries: Cherries, particularly tart cherries, have gained attention for their ability to reduce gout flares. They contain compounds that may help lower uric acid levels and ease joint pain....

Citrus Fruits: Vitamin C Boosters...

Citrus fruits like oranges, grapefruits, lemons, and limes are renowned for their vitamin C content. Vitamin C is a powerful antioxidant that can help quell inflammation and boost your immune system....

Oranges: Oranges are not only a great source of vitamin C but also provide fiber and potassium, which are beneficial for gout management....

Grapefruits: Grapefruits are loaded with antioxidants and provide hydration due to their high water content....

Lemons and Limes: These citrus fruits can add zesty flavor to your meals and beverages while providing vitamin C to combat inflammation....

Apples: Fiber for Gut Health...

The old adage "an apple a day keeps the doctor away" holds true when it comes to gout management. Apples are a good source of fiber, particularly soluble fiber called pectin. This fiber supports digestive health and helps regulate inflammation....

Incorporating Fruits Into Your Diet...

To harness the anti-inflammatory benefits of fruits, aim to incorporate a variety of them into your daily meals. Here are some practical tips:...

Fresh or Frozen: Fresh fruits are fantastic, but frozen fruits can be just as nutritious and convenient. Use them in smoothies, oatmeal, or as toppings for yogurt....

Snack Smart: Replace sugary snacks with whole fruits. They're not only satisfying but also provide long-lasting energy without the inflammation-triggering effects of refined sugar....

Salads and Salsas: Add fruits like berries or citrus segments to your salads or salsas for a burst of flavor and nutrition....

Homemade Desserts: When you have a sweet tooth, opt for homemade fruit-based desserts like berry crumbles or apple compotes instead of store-bought pastries....

In the following chapters, we will continue our exploration of anti-inflammatory foods, delving into vegetables, whole grains, lean proteins, nuts, seeds, and spices. By the time you finish this book, you'll have a wealth of knowledge and practical recipes to transform your diet and take control of your gout....

Chapter 6: Vegetables as Inflammation Fighters...

Vegetables are a cornerstone of any healthy diet, and they play a crucial role in combating inflammation associated with gout. In this chapter, we will explore a variety of vegetables that can be your allies in managing gout and achieving overall well-being....

Leafy Greens: A Nutrient-Rich Foundation...

Leafy greens like spinach, kale, Swiss chard, and collard greens are packed with vitamins, minerals, and antioxidants. They provide essential nutrients like folate and vitamin K while contributing to reduced inflammation....

Spinach: Spinach is a versatile leafy green that's high in antioxidants, especially vitamins A and C, which help combat inflammation....

Kale: Kale is a nutritional powerhouse containing vitamins K, A, and C, along with minerals like calcium and potassium. It's known for its anti-inflammatory properties....

Collard Greens: These greens are rich in fiber, vitamin C, and vitamin K. They are excellent for promoting gut health, which is vital for overall well-being....

Cruciferous Vegetables: Nature's Detoxifiers...

Cruciferous vegetables like broccoli, cauliflower, and Brussels sprouts contain compounds called glucosinolates, which can help detoxify the body and reduce inflammation....

Broccoli: Broccoli is a rich source of sulforaphane, a compound known for its anti-inflammatory and antioxidant properties....

Cauliflower: Cauliflower is versatile and can be used to create gout-friendly alternatives to high-purine foods, such as cauliflower rice or cauliflower crust pizza....

Colorful Vegetables: A Rainbow of Health...

Colorful vegetables like bell peppers, tomatoes, and carrots are not only visually appealing but also rich in antioxidants like beta-carotene and vitamin C, which help combat inflammation....

Bell Peppers: Bell peppers are an excellent source of vitamin C, providing a burst of flavor and health benefits to your meals....

Tomatoes: Tomatoes contain lycopene, an antioxidant that has been linked to reduced inflammation and a lower risk of gout attacks....

Preparing and Enjoying Vegetables...

Incorporating vegetables into your daily diet is a vital step toward gout management. Here are some practical tips for doing so:...

Salads: Create colorful salads with a mix of leafy greens, colorful vegetables, and lean proteins....

Stir-Fries: Prepare vegetable-packed stir-fries with tofu, chicken, or shrimp, using flavorful sauces and spices....

Roasting: Roast vegetables like broccoli, cauliflower, and bell peppers with a drizzle of olive oil and your favorite herbs and spices....

Soups and Stews: Add vegetables to soups and stews for added flavor, texture, and nutrition....

Smoothies: Blend leafy greens with fruits and a protein source like Greek yogurt for a nutrient-packed breakfast or snack....

As you continue your journey through this book, you'll discover even more ways to incorporate anti-inflammatory vegetables into your meals. Remember that variety is key to reaping the full spectrum of health benefits, so don't be afraid to try new vegetables and cooking techniques. Your taste buds and your joints will thank you....

Chapter 7: The Power of Whole Grains and Legumes...

In the quest for effective gout management through an anti-inflammatory diet, we turn our attention to whole grains and legumes. These nutrient-rich foods offer numerous health benefits, including the potential to reduce inflammation and support overall well-being....

Whole Grains: Nature's Nutrient Storehouse...

Whole grains are unprocessed grains that include the bran, germ, and endosperm. They are packed with essential nutrients, fiber, and antioxidants that can help combat inflammation....

Oats: Oats are an excellent source of soluble fiber, known for its anti-inflammatory properties. They can help lower levels of C-reactive protein, a marker of inflammation....

Quinoa: Quinoa is a complete protein, providing all nine essential amino acids. It's also rich in fiber, vitamins, and minerals, making it a superb choice for an anti-inflammatory diet....

Brown Rice: Brown rice is a whole grain that contains more nutrients and fiber than white rice. It can help stabilize blood sugar levels and reduce inflammation....

Legumes: Plant Protein Powerhouses...

Legumes, including beans, lentils, and chickpeas, are not only excellent sources of plant-based protein but also contain a variety of anti-inflammatory compounds....

Beans: Beans, such as black beans, kidney beans, and pinto beans, are high in fiber and antioxidants. They can help regulate blood sugar and reduce inflammation....

Lentils: Lentils are rich in protein, fiber, and various vitamins and minerals. They are a versatile addition to soups, stews, and salads....

Chickpeas: Chickpeas are not only the star of dishes like hummus but are also packed with protein and fiber that support a healthy inflammatory response....

Incorporating Whole Grains and Legumes...

Here are some practical tips for incorporating whole grains and legumes into your anti-inflammatory diet:...

Substitute: Swap refined grains (white bread, white rice) with whole grains (whole wheat bread, brown rice) to increase your fiber intake....

Salads and Soups: Add cooked lentils, chickpeas, or beans to salads and soups to boost protein and fiber content....

Grain Bowls: Create nutrient-dense grain bowls with quinoa,

brown rice, or barley as a base, and top with a variety of colorful vegetables and lean proteins....

Homemade Snacks: Roast chickpeas or create your own trail mix with whole grain cereals and nuts for a satisfying and anti-inflammatory snack....

Incorporating these whole grains and legumes into your diet not only provides essential nutrients but also contributes to the overall balance of your gout-friendly meals. As you continue to explore the chapters ahead, you'll gain a deeper understanding of how these foods can work in synergy with other anti-inflammatory ingredients to support your gout management journey....

Chapter 8: Lean Proteins for Gout Relief...

Protein is an essential macronutrient for overall health and well-being. However, when managing gout, it's crucial to choose lean protein sources that minimize the intake of purines, which can contribute to uric acid buildup. In this chapter, we'll explore various lean protein options that can play a pivotal role in gout relief....

The Importance of Lean Proteins...

Lean proteins are low in fat and purines, making them ideal choices for gout sufferers. They provide essential amino acids and can help maintain muscle mass and support overall health without exacerbating gout symptoms....

Poultry: Chicken and Turkey...

Chicken:...

Chicken is one of the most versatile and widely consumed lean proteins. It is low in purines and provides essential nutrients such as protein, vitamins, and minerals. Opt for skinless, boneless chicken breasts or thighs for the leanest cuts....

Turkey:...

Turkey is another excellent choice, especially lean turkey breast. It's rich in protein and provides essential amino acids without the risk of triggering gout attacks....

Fish: Omega-3 Rich Options...

Salmon:...

Salmon is a fatty fish rich in omega-3 fatty acids. Omega-3s have anti-inflammatory properties and can help reduce gout-related inflammation. Regular consumption of salmon can be beneficial for gout management....

Trout:...

Trout is another omega-3 rich fish that offers similar benefits. Grilled or baked trout can be a delicious and nutritious addition to your anti-inflammatory diet....

Plant-Based Proteins: Tofu and Legumes...

Tofu:...

Tofu, made from soybeans, is a versatile plant-based protein. It's low in purines and provides essential amino acids. Tofu can be used in various dishes, from stir-fries to smoothies....

Legumes:...

Beans, lentils, and chickpeas are not only excellent sources of plant-based protein but also contain fiber and antioxidants that promote anti-inflammatory effects. They can be used as a primary protein source or as complementary ingredients in various recipes....

Preparing Lean Proteins for Gout-Friendly Meals...

When preparing lean proteins for gout-friendly meals, consider these tips:...

Grilling and Baking: Grilling or baking chicken, turkey, or fish with herbs and spices can add flavor without adding excessive purines....

Marinades: Use low-purine marinades made from herbs, olive oil, and citrus juice to infuse flavor into lean proteins....

Portion Control: Be mindful of portion sizes to avoid overconsumption, as even lean proteins can contribute to uric acid production if consumed in excess....

Diverse Protein Sources: Incorporate a variety of lean protein sources into your diet to ensure a balanced intake of nutrients....

In the upcoming chapters, we will explore more anti-inflammatory ingredients and provide you with recipes that combine lean proteins with other gout-friendly foods. By making informed choices about your protein sources, you can take significant steps toward managing gout and reducing inflammation....

Chapter 9: Nuts and Seeds: Nature's Anti-Inflammatory Snacks...

When it comes to snacking on an anti-inflammatory diet for gout, nuts and seeds are your best friends. These small but mighty morsels are packed with healthy fats, antioxidants, and nutrients that can help reduce inflammation and support your overall health. In this chapter, we will explore a variety of nuts and seeds that can be incorporated into your gout-friendly diet....

Nuts: A Nutrient-Dense Powerhouse...

Nuts are nutrient-dense, offering an array of health benefits. They are rich in monounsaturated and polyunsaturated fats, which have been associated with reduced inflammation. Here are some nuts to consider:...

Almonds: Almonds are an excellent source of vitamin E, a

powerful antioxidant known for its anti-inflammatory properties. They also provide fiber and healthy fats....

Walnuts: Walnuts are high in omega-3 fatty acids, specifically alpha-linolenic acid (ALA). Omega-3s have been shown to reduce inflammation and may help with gout management....

Pistachios: Pistachios are a good source of protein, fiber, and antioxidants. They can be a satisfying and heart-healthy snack option....

Seeds: Tiny Nutritional Powerhouses...

Seeds are often overlooked but can be just as beneficial as nuts when it comes to fighting inflammation. They are rich in healthy fats, fiber, and essential nutrients. Here are some seeds to consider:...

Flaxseeds: Flaxseeds are renowned for their omega-3 content, particularly in the form of alpha-linolenic acid (ALA). Ground flaxseeds are more digestible and can be added to cereals, smoothies, or yogurt....

Chia Seeds: Chia seeds are packed with fiber, omega-3s, and antioxidants. They absorb liquid, creating a gel-like consistency that can help keep you feeling full and satisfied....

Pumpkin Seeds (Pepitas): Pumpkin seeds are a good source

of magnesium, which plays a role in muscle and nerve function. They are also rich in antioxidants like vitamin E and zinc....

Incorporating Nuts and Seeds Into Your Diet...

Nuts and seeds can be enjoyed in various ways as part of your anti-inflammatory diet:...

Snacking: Enjoy a handful of nuts or seeds as a satisfying and nutritious snack....

Smoothies: Blend nuts or seeds into your morning smoothie to add texture and flavor....

Salads: Sprinkle chopped nuts or seeds over salads for added crunch and nutrition....

Yogurt: Mix nuts or seeds into yogurt along with honey and fruit for a delicious and filling snack....

Baking: Incorporate nuts or seeds into baked goods like muffins, granola bars, or homemade bread for added nutrition....

By including a variety of nuts and seeds in your daily meals and snacks, you not only enhance the flavor and texture of your dishes but also provide your body with a wealth of anti-inflammatory nutrients. In the chapters to come, we will continue to explore anti-inflammatory ingredients and provide you with recipes that showcase the delicious possibilities of a gout-friendly diet....

Chapter 10: Herbs and Spices to Combat Gout Inflammation...

Herbs and spices are not just flavor enhancers; they are also powerful allies in the fight against inflammation. When used thoughtfully in your gout-friendly diet, these aromatic ingredients can add depth, complexity, and health benefits to your meals. In this chapter, we'll explore a range of herbs and spices known for their anti-inflammatory properties....

Turmeric: Nature's Anti-Inflammatory Gold...

Turmeric is a bright yellow spice derived from the root of the Curcuma longa plant. It contains an active compound called curcumin, which is a potent anti-inflammatory agent. Here's how you can incorporate turmeric into your diet:...

Golden Milk: Turmeric can be added to warm milk or milk alternatives to create a soothing drink known as golden milk. It's often sweetened with honey and spiced with black pepper for enhanced absorption....

Curries: Turmeric is a staple in many curry dishes, adding both color and flavor. Consider cooking up a delicious, gout-friendly vegetable curry with this spice....

Roasted Vegetables: Sprinkle turmeric over roasted vegetables like cauliflower or carrots to infuse them with its earthy flavor....

Ginger: A Zesty Anti-Inflammatory...

Ginger is a root known for its zesty and slightly sweet flavor. It contains gingerol, an active compound with anti-inflammatory and antioxidant properties. Here's how to use ginger:...

Tea: Ginger tea is a soothing beverage that can be made by steeping fresh ginger slices in hot water. Add a touch of honey or lemon for extra flavor....

Stir-Fries: Add grated or minced ginger to your stir-fry dishes for a burst of flavor and potential anti-inflammatory benefits....

Smoothies: Fresh or powdered ginger can be a spicy addition to your morning smoothie, pairing well with fruits like pineapple or mango....

Garlic: Flavorful and Anti-Inflammatory...

Garlic is not only a culinary superstar but also a potent anti-inflammatory ingredient. It contains allicin, a compound with potential anti-inflammatory properties. Here's how to incorporate garlic into your diet:...

Sauces and Dressings: Use minced garlic in homemade sauces, dressings, and marinades to add depth of flavor....

Roasted or Sautéed: Roast whole garlic bulbs or sauté minced garlic with vegetables to infuse your dishes with its savory taste....

Soups: Garlic can be a flavorful addition to soups and stews, enhancing both taste and nutrition....

Cinnamon: Sweet Spice with Health Benefits...

Cinnamon is a warm and sweet spice derived from the bark of trees. It contains antioxidants and has been linked to reduced inflammation. Here's how to enjoy cinnamon:...

Oatmeal: Sprinkle ground cinnamon on your morning oatmeal or cereal for added flavor and potential anti-inflammatory effects....

Baking: Use cinnamon in your baking recipes, such as muffins, pancakes, or homemade granola....

Beverages: Add a pinch of cinnamon to your coffee, tea, or smoothies for a warm, spicy twist....

As you explore the world of herbs and spices, remember that not only do they enhance the flavor of your meals, but they can also contribute to gout relief by reducing inflammation. In the upcoming chapters, we will continue to uncover the potential of anti-inflammatory foods and provide you with recipes that bring these ingredients to life in delicious and healthful ways....

Chapter 11: Hydration and Gout Management...

While it's essential to focus on anti-inflammatory foods, we must not overlook the role of proper hydration in gout management. Staying well-hydrated is a critical aspect of reducing the risk of gout attacks and supporting overall joint health. In this chapter, we'll delve into the relationship between hydration and gout and provide guidance on maintaining optimal fluid balance....

The Importance of Hydration...

Hydration plays several vital roles in gout management:...

Uric Acid Dilution:...

Adequate hydration helps dilute uric acid in the bloodstream, reducing the likelihood of uric acid crystal formation in the joints....

Joint Lubrication:...

Well-hydrated joints function more smoothly and experience less friction. Proper joint lubrication can help alleviate pain during gout attacks....

Kidney Function:...

The kidneys play a pivotal role in excreting excess uric acid from the body. When you're well-hydrated, your kidneys can work more effectively, lowering uric acid levels....

How Much Water Should You Drink?...

While the "eight glasses a day" rule is a common guideline, individual hydration needs can vary based on factors like climate, activity level, and overall health. A better approach is to pay attention to your body's signals:...

Thirst: Listen to your body. Thirst is a reliable indicator that it's time to drink water....

Urine Color: Pale yellow urine is a sign of good hydration, while dark yellow or amber urine may indicate dehydration....

Activity Level: If you're physically active or in a hot climate, you may need to drink more water to compensate for fluid loss through sweat....

Choosing Hydration Sources...

While water is the best choice for hydration, other fluids can contribute to your daily fluid intake:...

Herbal Teas: Unsweetened herbal teas, such as chamomile or mint, can be hydrating and provide additional anti-inflammatory benefits....

Infused Water: Add slices of cucumber, lemon, or berries to your water for a refreshing twist that encourages hydration....

Coconut Water: Coconut water is a natural source of electrolytes and can be a hydrating option, especially after physical activity....

Alcohol and Hydration...

Alcohol can dehydrate the body and increase the risk of gout attacks. If you choose to consume alcohol, do so in moderation and balance it with plenty of water to stay hydrated. Certain alcoholic beverages, such as beer and spirits, are more likely to trigger gout attacks, so be mindful of your choices....

Practical Hydration Tips...

Here are some practical tips for staying well-hydrated as part of your gout management plan:...

Carry a reusable water bottle with you to remind yourself to drink throughout the day....

Set hydration goals, such as drinking a glass of water before each meal....

Incorporate hydrating foods into your diet, such as watermelon, cucumbers, and celery....

Limit or avoid sugary and caffeinated beverages, as they can contribute to dehydration....

By maintaining proper hydration, you support your body's efforts to manage gout effectively and reduce the frequency and severity of gout attacks. In the upcoming chapters, we will continue to explore gout-friendly foods and lifestyle choices that work in harmony with hydration to promote your overall well-being....

Chapter 12: Weight Management for Gout Relief...

In the pursuit of gout relief and better overall health, maintaining a healthy weight is paramount. Excess body weight is closely linked to gout, as it can lead to higher uric acid levels and increase the risk of gout attacks. In this chapter, we'll explore the intricate connection between weight management and gout and provide practical guidance for achieving and maintaining a healthy weight....

The Weight-Gout Connection...

Gout and excess body weight
share a complex relationship:...

Uric Acid Production:...

Adipose tissue (body fat) produces
substances called cytokines, which
promote inflammation and can
increase uric acid production....

Uric Acid Clearance:...

Being overweight can impair the
kidneys' ability to excrete uric acid
efficiently, leading to higher uric
acid levels in the blood....

Joint Stress:...

Extra weight places added stress
on the joints, increasing the risk of
gout attacks and worsening joint
pain during flares....

Achieving and Maintaining a
Healthy Weight...

Achieving and maintaining a
healthy weight is crucial for gout
management. Here are some
strategies to help you reach your
weight goals:...

Balanced Diet:...

Adopt a balanced, calorie-
controlled diet that includes anti-
inflammatory foods, as discussed
in previous chapters. Pay attention
to portion sizes to prevent
overeating....

Regular Physical Activity:...

Engage in regular physical activity
to help with weight loss and
overall health. Low-impact
exercises like swimming, walking,

and cycling are gentle on the joints....

Gradual Progress:...

Aim for gradual, sustainable weight loss rather than quick fixes. Losing 1-2 pounds per week is a healthy and realistic goal....

Portion Control:...

Be mindful of portion sizes, especially when dining out. Ask for half-portions or share dishes to avoid overeating....

Hydration:...

Stay well-hydrated to support weight loss and maintain optimal kidney function....

The Role of Healthcare Professionals...

Consulting with a healthcare professional, such as a registered dietitian or a healthcare provider with expertise in gout management, can be immensely beneficial. They can help you develop a personalized weight management plan tailored to your unique needs and provide guidance on nutrition, exercise, and lifestyle changes....

Staying Committed to Your Goals...

Weight management is a long-term commitment that requires patience and perseverance. Keep in mind that achieving and maintaining a healthy weight is not just about managing gout; it's about improving your overall quality of life and reducing the risk of other chronic conditions....

In the subsequent chapters, we will continue to explore gout-friendly lifestyle choices, including exercise, stress management, and sleep, that contribute to your journey toward better gout control and overall well-being....

Chapter 13: Exercise for Gout Management and Joint Health...

Regular exercise is a crucial component of gout management and plays a pivotal role in maintaining overall joint health. Physical activity not only helps with weight management but also promotes improved joint function and reduced inflammation. In this chapter, we will explore the importance of exercise in gout relief and provide guidance on safe and effective workout routines....

The Benefits of Exercise for Gout...

Exercise offers a range of benefits for individuals with gout:...

Weight Management:...

Exercise helps burn calories, aiding in weight loss or weight maintenance, which is essential for gout management....

Joint Health:...

Regular movement helps maintain joint flexibility and can reduce the severity of gout attacks....

Improved Circulation:...

Physical activity enhances blood circulation, which can promote the removal of uric acid crystals from joints....

Reduced Inflammation:...

Exercise can have anti-inflammatory effects on the body, potentially reducing gout-related inflammation....

Enhanced Mood:...

Physical activity releases endorphins, which can help alleviate stress and improve your overall well-being....

Choosing the Right Exercise...

When it comes to exercise for gout management, the emphasis should be on low-impact activities that minimize stress on the joints. Here are some suitable options:...

Walking:...

Walking is a low-impact, accessible exercise that provides cardiovascular benefits and supports weight management....

Swimming and Water Aerobics:...

These exercises are gentle on the joints and offer resistance training for muscle strength....

Cycling:...

Cycling, whether on a stationary bike or outdoors, is an excellent way to improve cardiovascular fitness without joint stress....

Yoga and Stretching:...

Yoga and stretching exercises can enhance flexibility, balance, and joint mobility....

Strength Training:...

Light to moderate strength training with appropriate supervision can help build muscle, which supports joint stability....

Safety Considerations...

Before starting an exercise program, it's essential to consider your individual needs and any medical conditions. Here are some safety considerations for exercising with gout:...

Consult with a healthcare professional or physical therapist to create a personalized exercise plan....

Start slowly and gradually increase the intensity and duration of your workouts....

Pay attention to your body. If you experience pain or discomfort during exercise, stop and seek guidance....

Stay well-hydrated, especially during and after exercise, to prevent dehydration and reduce the risk of gout attacks....

Include warm-up and cool-down routines in your workouts to prepare your muscles and joints and prevent injury....

Staying Consistent...

Consistency is key to reaping the benefits of exercise for gout management. Aim for at least 150 minutes of moderate-intensity exercise per week, spread throughout the week. Remember that small, sustainable changes can make a significant difference in your overall health and gout relief....

In the following chapters, we will explore additional lifestyle choices, such as stress management and sleep, that can complement your exercise routine and contribute to your holistic approach to gout management and well-being....

Chapter 14: Stress Management for Gout Relief...

Stress is a common trigger for gout attacks and can exacerbate the symptoms of this painful condition. Learning effective stress management techniques is a valuable part of your gout management plan. In this chapter, we'll explore the connection between stress and gout, and we'll provide guidance on managing stress to reduce its impact on your health....

The Stress-Gout Connection...

Stress can contribute to gout in several ways:...

Uric Acid Production:...

Stress can stimulate the production of uric acid in the body, increasing the risk of gout attacks....

Immune Response:...

Stress can weaken the immune system, making it less effective at managing inflammation....

Lifestyle Factors:...

Stress can lead to unhealthy coping mechanisms such as poor dietary choices, alcohol consumption, and lack of physical activity, all of which can trigger gout attacks....

Stress Management Techniques...

Effective stress management can help reduce the risk of gout attacks and improve your overall well-being. Here are some stress management techniques to consider:...

Mindfulness Meditation:...

Mindfulness meditation can help you stay present, reduce anxiety, and manage stress effectively. It involves focusing your attention on the present moment and accepting it without judgment....

Deep Breathing:...

Practicing deep breathing exercises can calm your nervous system and reduce stress. Try inhaling deeply through your nose for a count of four, holding your breath for four counts, and exhaling slowly through your mouth for four counts....

Progressive Muscle Relaxation:...

Progressive muscle relaxation involves tensing and then relaxing different muscle groups in your body. This practice can release physical tension and promote relaxation....

Physical Activity:...

Regular exercise is an excellent way to reduce stress. Engage in activities you enjoy, such as walking, swimming, or yoga, to help alleviate stress....

Stress-Reduction Techniques:...

Explore stress-reduction techniques such as journaling, art therapy, or spending time in nature to find what works best for you....

Social Support:...

Talking to friends, family members, or a therapist can

provide emotional support and help you manage stress....

Lifestyle Changes for Stress Reduction...

In addition to specific stress management techniques, consider making lifestyle changes that promote relaxation and overall well-being:...

Prioritize Sleep: Aim for quality sleep by establishing a regular sleep schedule and creating a relaxing bedtime routine....

Balanced Diet: Maintain a gout-friendly diet rich in anti-inflammatory foods to support overall health and minimize dietary triggers....

Limit Alcohol and Caffeine: Reduce or eliminate alcohol and caffeine, which can contribute to stress and disrupt sleep patterns....

Time Management: Prioritize tasks and set realistic goals to reduce the pressure of overwhelming schedules....

Creating a Stress-Resistant Lifestyle...

Stress is a part of life, but it's essential to manage it effectively to support your gout management efforts. By incorporating stress management techniques and making lifestyle changes, you can create a stress-resistant lifestyle that promotes gout relief and improves your overall quality of life....

In the final chapter, we will explore the importance of sleep in gout management and provide tips for achieving restful and restorative sleep....

Chapter 15: The Role of Sleep in Gout Management...

Quality sleep is a fundamental aspect of gout management and overall well-being. Poor sleep patterns can not only trigger gout attacks but also exacerbate the pain and inflammation associated with this condition. In this final chapter, we will explore the connection between sleep and gout, and we'll provide practical tips for achieving restful and restorative sleep....

The Sleep-Gout Connection...

The relationship between sleep and gout is complex:...

Uric Acid Metabolism:...

Sleep plays a crucial role in the regulation of uric acid metabolism. Poor sleep patterns can lead to increased uric acid levels in the bloodstream....

Inflammation:...

Chronic sleep deprivation can promote systemic inflammation, exacerbating gout-related inflammation and joint pain....

Pain Sensitivity:...

Lack of sleep can lower your pain threshold, making gout attacks feel more intense and painful....

Tips for Restful Sleep...

To improve the quality of your sleep and support gout management, consider the following tips:...

Consistent Sleep Schedule:...

Go to bed and wake up at the same time every day, even on weekends, to regulate your body's internal clock....

Create a Relaxing Bedtime Routine:...

Engage in calming activities before bed, such as reading, gentle stretching, or taking a warm bath....

Comfortable Sleep Environment:...

Ensure your bedroom is dark, quiet, and cool. Invest in a comfortable mattress and pillows....

Limit Screen Time:...

Reduce exposure to screens (phones, tablets, computers, TVs) at least an hour before bedtime, as the blue light emitted can interfere with sleep....

Watch Your Diet:...

Avoid heavy meals, caffeine, and alcohol close to bedtime. Opt for a light, gout-friendly snack if needed....

Exercise Regularly:...

Engaging in regular physical activity can promote better sleep.

However, avoid vigorous exercise close to bedtime....

Manage Stress:...

Use stress management techniques discussed in previous chapters to alleviate anxiety and promote relaxation before sleep....

Limit Naps:...

While short naps can be rejuvenating, long or late-day naps can disrupt nighttime sleep. Keep naps to 20-30 minutes and earlier in the day....

Consulting a Healthcare Professional...

If you continue to experience sleep disturbances despite making these adjustments, consider consulting a healthcare professional. Sleep disorders, such as sleep apnea or insomnia, can contribute to poor sleep quality and may require specific interventions or treatments....

Prioritizing Sleep for Gout Relief...

Quality sleep is a pillar of gout management. By implementing these tips and adopting a sleep-friendly lifestyle, you can reduce the risk of gout attacks, alleviate inflammation, and enhance your overall quality of life. A holistic approach to gout management, encompassing dietary choices, exercise, stress management, and sleep, can empower you to take control of your gout and enjoy a more pain-free and fulfilling life....

In closing, remember that gout management is a journey, and the choices you make each day can have a profound impact on your health and well-being. By incorporating the knowledge and strategies from this book into your life, you are taking meaningful steps toward gout relief and a healthier future....